I0420738

Ageless Beauty

100+ Beauty Tips and Regimens For A Glowing And Healthy Skin

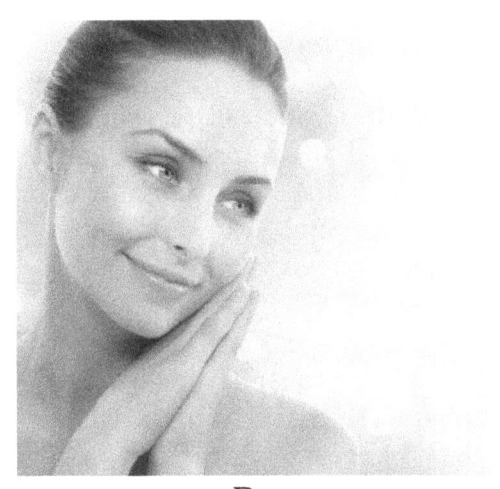

By
Fhilcar Faunillan

Fhilcar Faunillan

Copyright 2015 by Content Arcade Publishing - All rights reserved.

This document is geared towards providing exact and reliable information in regards to the topic and issue covered. The publication is sold with the idea that the publisher is not required to render accounting, officially permitted, or otherwise, qualified services. If advice is necessary, legal or professional, a practiced individual in the profession should be ordered.

- From a Declaration of Principles which was accepted and approved equally by a Committee of the American Bar Association and a Committee of Publishers and Associations.

In no way is it legal to reproduce, duplicate, or transmit any part of this document in either electronic means or in printed format. Recording of this publication is strictly prohibited and any storage of this document is not allowed unless with written permission from the publisher. All rights reserved.

The information provided herein is stated to be truthful and consistent, in that any liability, in terms of inattention or otherwise, by any usage or abuse of any policies, processes, or directions contained within is the solitary and utter responsibility of the recipient reader. Under no circumstances will any legal responsibility or blame be held against the publisher for any reparation, damages, or monetary loss due to the information herein, either directly or indirectly.

Respective authors own all copyrights not held by the publisher.

The information herein is offered for informational purposes solely, and is universal as so. The presentation of the information is without contract or any type of guarantee assurance.

The trademarks that are used are without any consent, and the publication of the trademark is without permission or backing by the trademark owner. All trademarks and brands within this book are for clarifying purposes only and are the owned by the owners themselves, not affiliated with this document.

Table of Contents

INTRODUCTION

I want to thank you and congratulate you for downloading the book, *"Ageless Beauty: 100 Beauty Tips And Regimens For A Glowing And Healthy Skin"*.

Your skin is one of the largest organs of your body that holds you apiece and keeps your first-hand protection from many chemicals that you get exposed to. It is one of the parts that people will immediately see when they see you. And you cannot deny it, people can make an impression out of you by just looking at your skin since it is the layer that reflects the healthiness of your inner body as well. Thus, the need to take good care of it should be a must—not merely for convenience or fads but for habits to keep your skin healthy and glowing.

There are many aspects in which you can target when you decide to have a healthier skin. You can reframe your diet and opt for healthier foods with those that have beneficial effects on the skin. You can also improve on your sanitation habits. Or if you are into skin care cosmetic products, you may also want to invest on those that are effective and safe to use. Or if you are money-pincher, you might want to find cheaper and more natural alternatives of skin care products and actually make your own. You can take any approach that you want as long as you keep these factors working for your inner and outer glow.

Your skin may be prone to different problems such as skin cancer, psoriasis, eczema, or even more common ones like acne—blackheads and white heads. These can usually affect the face, neck, back, chest, and shoulders. However, with proper care and healthy regimens, these skin problems may be avoided and may even flip over to give you the chance of having beautiful, glowing, and younger-looking skin that is healthy, both inside and out.

Thanks again for downloading this book, I hope you enjoy it!

Chapter 1 - All About Your Skin

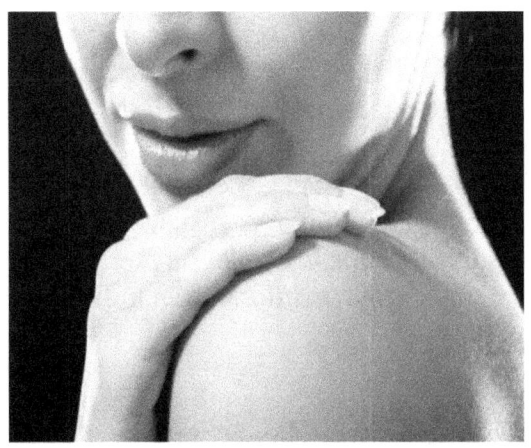

Our skin serves many purposes in your body. Sometimes we take it for granted that we do not really mind what we do and how it actually affects our skin. But for some reminding, our skin needs care and attention for these following reasons:

Our First-Hand Protective Barrier

We expose ourselves to many particles every single day when we go out for work, school, or even just to spend some leisure time outdoors or indoors. Anywhere we go, our skin interacts with all the chemicals it gets to rub and encounter with in the atmosphere. The skin mainly protects us from all the harmful effects that these particles can bring by serving as the first layer of interaction. If this first barrier gets damaged, these chemicals may immediately affect our organs inside and may dangerously cause further damage that will be more difficult to handle.

An Outlet of Toxic Wastes from Our Body

Our skin may release the toxins in our body through sweating. This release aids the body in getting rid of all the wastes in the system for organs to function well. Without the skin as an outlet for these toxic wastes, they may clump up and accumulate inside our bodies and cause harm to our internal organs. Our skin's ability to perspire makes it an essential part of keeping our insides free of problems.

Can be a Diagnostic Tool

Our skin can be a body condition barometer. Many internal problems manifest on the skin as well, giving us warning signs that something wrong is going on inside our system. Without this function of the skin, internal problems may worsen without our knowledge that they can no longer be tended. The way our skin reflects our insides makes it an important window to the health of the whole body.

Provide Us Comfort

Whatever the weather condition may be, our skin is the very first part that gets exposed to it. And depending on how cold or hot it is, our skin and body adjust pretty well just to provide us with the kind of comfort that we need. When it is cold, our skin triggers shivers down our spine, causing the body to generate heat. And when we feel hot, we perspire to cool down the body's temperature. In short, our skin provides us with comfort whatever the weather is to keep our systems in balance.

Provide Us with Pleasure

With the sense of touch, we feel pleasure through our skin. It is what often hold bonds together, such as familial, friendly, and intimate relationships. From simple brushing of the skin, to holding hands, to warm hugs, and more, our skin gives us the ability to feel pleasure.

Chapter 2 - Food For A Healthier Skin

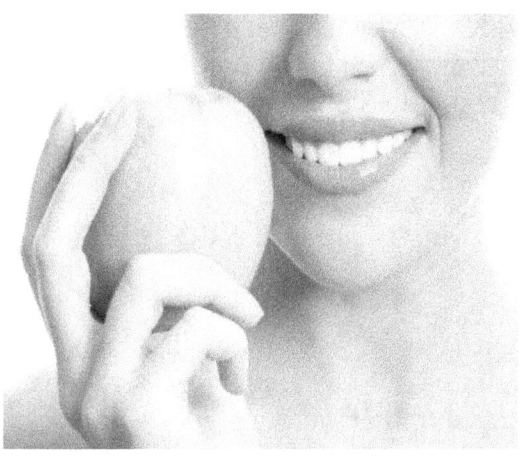

The common adage, *we are what we eat,* makes no room for exemption when it comes to our skin. Whatever food we take inside our system gets reflected on our skin. If you feed yourself with healthy food, you will most likely have a healthy and younger-looking skin as compared to when you munch mostly on junk food.

You skin needs nutrients from what you eat. And like every other organ, it absorbs these nutrients to use for its constant functioning. When the nutrients that goes

23

into your skin could not suffice, your skin may look dry, scaly, wrinkled, and becomes prone to skin problems like acne, or worse skin cancer.

Which is why it is very important for you to watch what you eat to see how it affects your skin.

Skin Care Tip #1: Nuts Are Not NOTS

Mixed nuts such as Brazilian nuts, walnuts, and macadamias are high in nutrients that can help your skin become healthier. Brazilian nuts have high selenium content which is an essential substance in increasing the skin's elasticity and decreasing the chances of skin cancer. Walnuts are also rich in omega-3 fatty acids that can aid the lessening of skin inflammation and cracking. And lastly, macadamias are also rich in healthy oil and fatty acids that can rejuvenate the skin. With a mix of these three, you can achieve a healthier looking skin.

Skin Care Tip #2: Do not take the Dairy dare

Organic or not, dairy products contain cow hormones that cause your oil glands on your pores to activate highly. This stimulation may lead to the formation of acne and of course, a healthy skin does not involve having acne. So, you might have to give up the consumption of excess dairy products.

Skin Care Tip #3: Opt for Watermelon as a snack

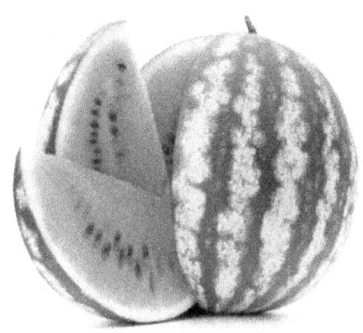

The pinkish flesh of the watermelon can provide you with lycopene which can reduce and buffer the harsh effects of the sun on your skin. It helps lessen the redness and damage caused by the sun on your skin. It prevents your skin from wrinkling and it lowers your risk of skin cancer.

Skin Care Tip #4: Drink plenty of water

Water is the basic body cleaner. It can clear off the toxins on your skin that usually causes the blemishes and inflammations. Water also aids in the transportation of the nutrients and oxygen to the skin to prevent it from dehydration or drying up. In a cheap stake of water consumption, you can already step up in keeping your skin healthy.

Skin Care Tip #5: Deep-fried, a no-no

Ditch the pack French Fries or that one piece of extra spicy fried chicken dipped in a sea of boiling lard. Food which are high in fats and carbs like them will cause your skin to wrinkle. Instead, stick to a cleaner diet to have a cleaner and clearer skin.

Skin Care Tip #6: Eat up your vegetables

Never ever skip on eating that vegetable side-dish or that vegetable salad. As much as possible, throw in vegetables in every meal that you consume every single day. Vegetables are rich in antioxidant free-radicals, nutrients, and anticancer properties that keeps the skin healthy and of lower cancer risk.

Skin Care Tip #7: Citrus fruits are your friends

As much as Vitamin C holds the immune system's strength, it can also mop up the free radicals that cause your skin to wrinkle and sag. With the consumption of more citrus fruits, you are eliminating the toxins and thus keeping your skin healthy looking and have that healthy feeling.

Skin Care Tip #8: Berry is good for your Skin

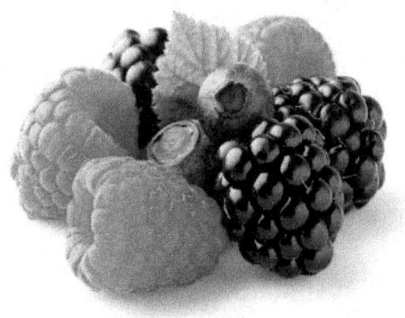

Throw in some berries into your smoothies or meals. They are rich in *ellagic acid* which are high in antioxidants that prevent your skin from wrinkling. Ellagic acid protects the skin's collagen to keep it younger looking and plump.

Skin Care Tip #9: Cut on Carbs

Carbohydrates will increase the insulin level in your system. With a red alert of insulin level, a dullness of your skin lingers. It will cause it to look dry and wrinkly. Carbohydrates may be consumed since it still is a source of energy but if it is taken in excess, its adverse effects on your skin will show.

Skin Care Tip #10: Healthy Fats

Fats are not scary as long as they are in modicum amount and most especially when the fats you are consuming are healthy. Opt for avocadoes, nuts, and other food with healthy fats to keep the dullness of the skin away and to make it appear healthy inside and out. Avoid those trans-fats.

Skin Care Tip #11: Reduce Sugar Consumption

The sweetness of sugar may seem like a traitor to our skin's health for it causes damage to the skin's collagen and elastin, which may lead to having wrinkles. So, as much as possible, reduce your sugar consumption.

Skin Care Tip #12: Cleanse and Detoxify Your Way Out

The toxins inside your body can cause damage to the skin cells that may further cause your skin to age fast. Detoxifying through cleansing juices may save up the process and will help you have a younger-looking skin.

Skin Care Tip #13: More Fiber Inside for Outer Glow

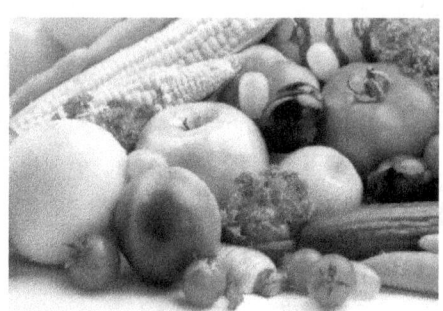

Some skin problems and impurities are only caused by digestive problems. With proper nutrition, your skin will glow into its full blown health. Fiber can help in removing toxins from the body, making way for nutrients to get transferred efficiently and effectively. So, boost up your diet with more fiber and detoxify from within for a noticeable glow outside.

Skin Care Tip #14: Cold Raw Milk for Your Skin

For a softer, more glowing and radiant skin, you may engage in a morning ritual of washing your face with cold and raw milk. This will instantly freshen up your face and improve your skin tone and complexion. You may also choose to add cucumber juice to the milk. Use a cotton ball and wipe it on your face.

Skin Care Tip #15: Coffee as a natural exfoliator

Coffee grounds will not only keep you awake but they can also awaken the renewal process of your skin. As natural exfoliators, theses can help in getting rid of dead skin cells, making it look healthier and more radiant.

Skin Care Tip #16: Skip on Sodium

If you accumulate all the sodium that you have consumed from your processed foods, you might get a little scared on how it affects your skin. Too much sodium consumption may lead to puffiness on the areas around the eyes and jawline puffy. Processed foods such as canned goods, packed noodles, and almost anything that went through factory packing and mixing contain sodium. Instead of these products, you may opt for healthier foods such as fruits and vegetables.

Skin Care Tip #17: Make Iron your Fuel

Pumping more iron into your system does not only improve your blood but your skin condition too. It gives you the payoff of having plumper, more toned, and firmer skin up from the neck down to the lower muscles. It helps you get rid of saggy skin, thus making you look younger.

Skin Care Tip #18: Tea as Skin Safeguards

Tea, most especially green and black tea, can help prevent skin cancer and wrinkles as it fights against the collagen breakdown. These teas have compounds called EGCG and *theaflavins* that act as guardians of the skin, protecting it from skin problems.

Skin Care Tip #19: Eat Your Way to a Healthier Skin

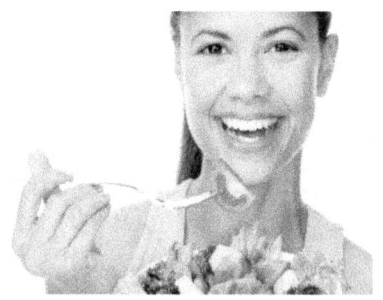

Eat your way to a healthier skin. As much as possible, throw in some carrots into your meals every single day. Carrots are rich in Retin-A which help reduce the stress-caused fine lines around your eyes.

Skin Care Tip #20: Garnish Your Food with Parsley

Parsley's high sebum balancing property makes it a great treatment for skin blemishes like acne. Parsley can get rid of the toxins on the skin by unclogging the pores. Acne breakouts and other skin problems are reduced. So, as much as possible, top your food with parsley and enjoy your share of it as well.

Skin Care Tip #21: Sardines for Your Skin

These little creatures in a bunch are rich in a type of omega-3 known as DHA. This has an anti-inflammatory property that can reduce the breakout of acne. Acne is mainly caused by inflammation but with the addition of sardines in your diet, your risk in developing these blemishes becomes relatively lower.

Skin Care Tip #22: Throw in Some Kale

Kale is high in *lutein* and *zeaxanthin* that can help in taking in and neutralizing the free radicals given off by UV rays. Even when you have applied sunscreen, some wavelengths may still get through your protection. A cup of kale a day can actually provide you with the benefits of having firmer skin along with additional Vitamins C and A in your skin.

Skin Care Tip #23: Almond Milk for a Healthier Skin

You can have milk that is not under the dairy category. Almond milk is rich in anti-inflammatory properties that can fight off acne breakouts, wrinkles, and rashes. If you cannot give up drinking milk, at least have the unsweetened almond milk for a healthier skin.

Skin Care Tip #24: Taste Some Oysters

Oysters have high zinc content that can help in the growth and development of skin cells. In some studies, oyster consumption can actually reduce chances of having blemishes such as whiteheads and blackheads.

Skin Care Tip #25: Always have Some Spice

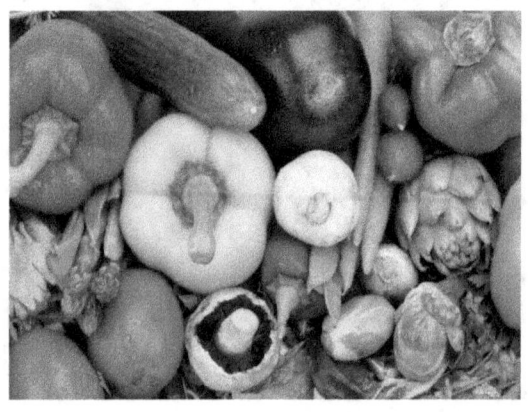

Yellow bell peppers are rich in antioxidants that can fight off the free radicals on the skin that cause evident signs of aging like wrinkling. This spice does not only make our food taste and smell better but works for the skin's health as well. So do not skip yellow bell peppers, they are actually healthy for your skin.

Skin Care Tip #26: Kiwi Benefits

Kiwi has wallops of Vitamin C that does not only protect the immune system but also stimulates the synthesis of collagen on the skin which makes it appear firmer and smoother. Kiwi's richness in Vitamin C is associated with having lesser wrinkles and cracking of the skin.

Skin Care Tip #27: Consume Pumpkin-Based Recipes

Pumpkins are high in bet-carotene that is transformed into Vitamin A by the body. Vitamin A is used in the growth of the skin cells, thus making the skin look smoother, fresher, and softer. So, whatever kind of pumpkin recipe you choose —whether you want pies or casseroled pumpkins, you can have the benefits of the beta-carotene.

Skin Care Tip #28: Have a Sip of Classic Red Wine

Studies show that adults who had *actinic keratoses*, a form of skin lesion caused by continuous exposure to the sun's harsh rays, has lowered their condition state by 28% when they sipped half a glass of red wine every day. This is perhaps due to the *resvatrol* content of red wine that is an antioxidant with anti-tumor forming properties.

Skin Care Tip #29: Sunflower Seeds for a Brighter Skin

One of the sources of Vitamin E that is necessary for prevention of skin blemishes are sunflower seeds. The lower your Vitamin E levels are, the more potential you have to develop pimples and acnes. Vitamin E helps your body fight against inflammation that can lead to these skin problems. So, you can snack and munch on some sunflower seeds for a healthier source of skin nutrients.

Skin Care Tip #30: Bean There, Still There

Foods high in glycemic content can increase blood sugar or insulin levels that can cause hormonal changes that lead to acne. So, for a blemish-free skin, you might want to include beans like chickpeas in your meals. These beans are low in glycemic content and are, instead, rich in fiber and protein that can slow down the body's digestive process and sugar response. Protein also aids in skin cell production giving your skin a healthier glow.

Chapter 3 - Your Skin and Its Environment

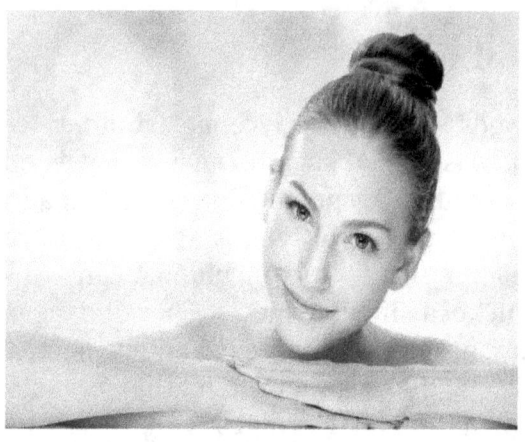

No matter how much you feed your insides with healthy food, your skin will need its support from the outside as well. Having a clean environment will help in improving the health of your skin as it always will be exposed to the particles present around you.

The particles like dust and other harmful substances that you may not know of can create a reaction on your skin and if it does not favor the particles, then you are up to an unfavorable irritation and rashes, or worse even a development of some serious skin problems. Given that reason, it is very important for you to watch for your environment and how it may affect the health of your skin, most especially that, more or less, you can have a sense of control over your surroundings.

Skin Care Tip #31: Keep a clean space

No matter how much you feed yourself with healthy food, they can only do so much fighting when the environment you are exposed to will not aid in the full bloom of your skin. Keep a clean space — from your room, down to your kitchen, living room, and the other rooms of the house, from the biggest appliance down to the smallest ornament. Make sure they are out of dust and other toxins that make irritate your skin. Once it gets irritated, it can be prone to further damage.

Skin Care Tip #32: Keep your make-up brushes clean

Sometimes we rush in applying our make-up that we end up stashing our brushes away without cleaning them. See to it that every after using your brush, you keep it off with the cosmetics that you used it on. If these chemicals stay in your brush from the last time you used them, they will mix up with the chemicals that you will use now. Some of these reactions can irritate your skin and can cause infections, inflammations, and blemishes. So to avoid them, make it a habit to clean your make-up brushes after you use them.

Skin Care Tip #33: Sanitize your mobile phones

Do you remember all the places that you have left your cellphone at – the table, floor, or that empty chair where no one was seated? Basically, we carry our mobile phones anywhere and leave it temporarily in a place where it is convenient for us to pick it up again. The amount of germs our mobile phones have will keep us close to having infections on the skin as well as irritations and inflammations. These viruses and germs may cause damage to the skin that will keep it from becoming healthier and younger looking.

Skin Care Tip #34: Do not wear make-up to bed

Never go to sleep without washing your make-up off of your face. If you do so, your pores will clog up and this may cause breakouts on your skin. When our pores clog up, serum, which is a waxy lubricant that helps moisturize our skin cells, will fail to do its job thus making the skin more prone to dryness and cracking. Moreover, serum builds up inside and may already cause acne. So, thoroughly wash off your face of the make-up or you may also use a make-up remover to get rid of the chemicals right before you divulge into a peaceful slumber.

Skin Care Tip #35: Hands off of your face

The culprit right behind the acne on your skin lies at the tips of your fingers. Your hands may have grazed a lot of items right before you touch your face. And even without realizing it, you just delivered bacteria like p. acne to your skin. This may trigger an acne breakout. So as much as possible, if you know your hands are dirty, keep them off your face. But if you cannot help yourself from keeping your hands off your skin, at least make sure they are clean right before you do so.

Skin Care Tip #36: Exfoliate Effortlessly

Your skin has its natural way of exfoliating. When you hurry yourself with the process and apply methods using your bare hands, you may cause problems on your skin, instead. So, do not force your skin to exfoliate under pressure. You may do so using other skin care products or homemade products but do not ever put the decision and action at the very tips of your fingers.

Skin Care Tip #37: Limit bath time

Long baths and showers may remove the natural moisturizers on your skin. Without these natural oils, your skin will dry and may easily get irritated. So, you may just want to limit your bath time — you are not only conserving water, you are also saving your skin from harm.

Skin Care Tip #38: Pat dry instead of scrubbing

After taking a bath, showering, or even just washing a part of your body, gently pat your skin with a towel instead of rubbing it. Scrubbing can lead to drying off the moisture on your skin while simply patting it would help retain moisture.

Skin Care Tip #39: Invest on Dry Brushing

Dry brushing is a simple skin care that is cheap and gives you a multitude of benefits. It helps in eliminating the dead cells on your skin to make room for new and younger looking skin; gets rid of cellulites; stimulates your hormones; and even tightens the skin for a better circulation and nutrient and oxygen transportation. So you may invest on a great skin brush and experience all these benefits on your skin.

Skin Care Tip #40: Never ever put the extraction duties on your hands

Removing your blackheads with your bare hands may lead you to having cyst formation, scarring, breaking, and other skin infections. This kind of extraction can damage the tissues around the area with black heads. The black heads may be removed but the tissues have been damaged already.

Skin Care Tip #41: Give Your Skin a Breather, Have a No Make-Up Day

Adding up make-up on your skin every single day means you are putting on chemicals that are clogging up your pores. When you clog them up constantly, you are taking a closer step towards more skin problems such as skin cancer, permanent skin discoloration, and even allergies and other unusual skin reactions. So, allow your pores to breathe and go on for a no make-up day. Surely, still you would not look any less beautiful than you are.

Skin Care Tip #42: Wax over Shave

Although shaving can cause you to have smoother and clearer skin, it is still very much harmful, especially when you compare it to waxing. Opt for hot wax instead of shaving when you clear off your skin hair. Hot wax is a lot gentler on your skin than the shaving process.

Skin Care Tip #43: Learn to Let Go of Your Products

You may have make-up products that have changed in color and odor or mascaras that have hardened enough that they do not serve their purpose any longer. When your products look like these, accept the fact that they now belong in the garbage can. Throw out these products because if you still use them in your skin, they may cause irritation and infection.

Skin Care Tip #44: Own your Make-Up Products

You may share your blessings but not your make-up. As much as possible, for hygiene purposes, keep your make-up products for personal use. Certain reactions and transfer of bacteria may cause some blemish breakage.

Skin Care Tip #45: Be Careful With Tattoo Needles

You have to be careful with tattoo needles, not only with the reason that they prick but because of hygienic purposes as well. When needles used in tattoo-making are not properly cleaned, they may pass on infections directly, especially that these tattoos and colored inks are inserted right under your skin.

Skin Care Tip #46: Love Your Hands, Wear your Gloves

Your hands work hard enough in cleaning and more so, they get exposed to chemicals in soaps, acids, and other cleaning products that make them prone to damage. So, love your hands and keep them smooth and soft by wearing your rubber gloves when you clean.

Chapter 4- Your Skin and the Science of Cosmetics

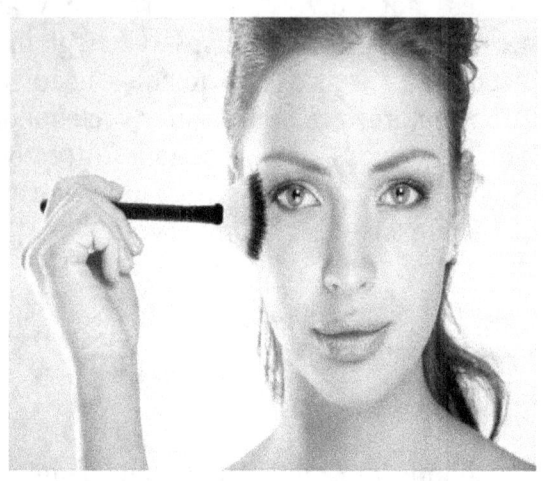

Stress is felt when a person feels like one is incapable of achieving a certain goal. Well, imagine not just feeling incapable but actually being incapable of doing something you desire to do. That is a whole lot of stress you have on your already-filled plate.

With the rise of technology, researchers — dermatologists and scientists, have discovered new methods on how to improve ways on taking care of the skin. With a combination of a few chemicals that would tend to what the customers need, they could expect effective and successful results. There are many cosmetic products that are said to be effective and already proven to be safe as well. However, there are also those that still need your double attention.

Using cosmetics for a healthier skin is not an entire no-no, it is merely in between a yes and no. All you have to be extra careful with what you use. Make sure that the product has been well-tested and safe to use because in worst case scenarios, instead of having better-looking skin and solving skin problems, they might just give you skin problems.

Skin Care Tip #47: Keep Your Skin Care Products Simple

The simpler your skin care products are, the safer you are from skin irritation and infection. Remember that these products differently contain chemicals and a mixture of all of them may not be of your liking. Worse, it would cause your skin redness, breakage, and other skin diseases. In choosing your skin care products, the simpler they are, the better.

Skin Care Tip #48: Follow the Make-up Sequence

In applying make-up, it is best to start off with the thinnest application then towards the rougher and more powdered ones. Start off with the concealer or baby cream upon applying make-up.

Skin Care Tip #49: Invest on a good and reliable sunscreen

Sunscreens should be basics in your skin care kit. With the present climatic conditions, you will need stronger and more reliable protection from the sun. So, do not thrift up your money on buying a sunscreen. Invest on good quality and tested sunscreens.

Skin Care Tip #50: Start with a Blank Slate

Before applying any cosmetic product on your face, make sure that you have washed it off already and patted it dry. Start off with your face clean since you do not want to add make-up that can clog up your pores when you know that your pores still have particles that may get stuck there. So, make sure that even before applying the basic firsts in make-up, you have already washed your face.

Skin Care Tip #51: Moisturize your Skin

A lot of skin problems start off with a dry skin. Washing off your face into squeaky clean results only says that you have dried up your skin well. However, this cleanliness does not necessarily mean your skin is already healthy. When your skin is dry, you are under the recipe of further skin problems such as cracking and breaking that may lead to irritation and inflammation. So add up trusted brands of moisturizers on your skin and do not leave it with further skin issues.

Skin Care Tip #52: Apply Sunscreen with SPF 15 or higher

With too much sun, your skin might get damaged — dry and at risk for skin cancer. To keep this from happening, do not forget to apply sunscreen on your skin with at least an SPF of 15. You may smother yourself with it and reapply every two hours, most especially when you are continuously staying under the bashing heat of the sun.

Skin Care Tip #53: Give up the Strong Soaps

Strong detergents and body soaps may strip off the natural oils from your skin.

Skin Care Tip #54: Save through Shaving

Shaving is okay if done correctly. Keep your skin protected by lubricating your skin before shaving — you may apply shaving cream, gel, or lotion then use a clear, clean, and sharp razor. You may already shave in the direction of your hair and not against it.

Skin Care Tip #55: The irony of heavy-duty cleansers

Avoid heavy-duty skin care products. Many of these chemicals will rub off your skin squeaky clean. But despite the nil presence of bacteria that they promise you, they also rip off your skin's moisture which keeps your skin more prone to infections.

Skin Care Tip #56: Water-based and oil-Free for Acne Prone Skin

If you know you are prone to having acne, you may want to lessen in application of your moisturizing products on your skin. Doing so may only cause breakout. Instead, use oil-free and water-based moisturizers.

Skin Care Tip #57: Consider Using Petroleum Jelly

Petroleum jelly is a cheap and common product that actually has many uses for the skin. It can serve as a moisturizer for those skin parts that are cracking — feet, elbows, hands, lips, cuticles, nails, and others. It can also protect your skin from chafing when you are wearing a new pair of shoes, or going out for a run or cycle. It can also cool down a few scrapes and bumps on your skin and be used as an ointment as well. Petroleum jelly is a product that you can really invest on when you want to take care of your skin. It is inexpensive but it can guarantee you many effective uses.

Skin Care Tip #58: Invest on Dual-Functioning Skin Care Products

There are cosmetics that can give you more effect in just one application. You may want to invest on these products as it means applying lesser chemicals on your skin and saving on skin care product budget.

Skin Care Tip #59: Expensive and Effective not Exclusive

In using your cosmetic products, you have to bear in mind that not all expensive products can guarantee you successful and safe effects. There are certain products that are expensive that will only cause you further costs because they may lead to infections and other skin problems.

Skin Care Tip #60: Moisturize your Skin

It is not enough to just have your skin clean and exfoliated, keeping it moisturized also reflects its healthiness. With the right moisturizer for your skin, you may have less chances of having dry skin that is the main ingredient for further skin problems such as deep lines and skin cancer. Moisturizers may provide you with additional skin care protection.

Skin Care Tip #61: Go Scream for Eye Cream

There is an area on our faces that we almost never really get to touch and have time to care of: the areas around our eyes. They often appear black and saggy most especially when we are stressed. But just like every other skin area, these parts also deserve some care and loving. Some eye cream application on the said areas may reduce creases and crinkles that form under your eyes. Dab it gently on the edge of your bones surrounding the eyes and spread slowly.

Skin Care Tip #62: Lip Protection

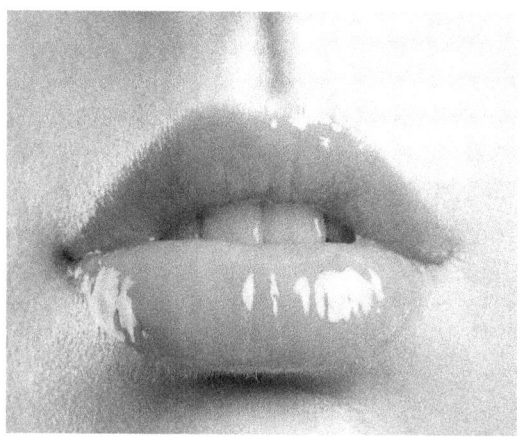

Your lips is among those skin areas which is prone to dryness, cracking, bleeding, and other injuries because of its thinness and lack of oil glands that normally keeps the skin naturally moist. So with that, you need to pay attention to your lips and actually take good care of it, most especially when you are constantly exposed to the sun and stress. With these risks, you are more prone to having lips that can easily be wounded. In order to reduce these problems, you may apply lip balm with SPF or petroleum jelly regularly.

Skin Care Tip #63: Make Sure your Skin Care Products and Your Skin are Destined

Even in cosmetic use, you may still need some match-making. There are products that will not suit your skin and there are products that will cause your skin to glow effectively. Your duty is to find the products that will work best for you, not give you further problems.

Skin Care Tip #64: Have a Milk of Magnesia Facial

For softer and more glowing skin, apply a milk of magnesia facial. Make sure your hands are clean before putting on the facial and applying it on your face. Leave it on your skin for 5 to 10 minutes and afterwards, cleanse it off with warm water.

Skin Care Tip #65: Read Skin Care Product Labels

Much like reading food labels, you should also learn how to read the labels of skin care products. Some of the ingredients may just swerve you out of your purpose and cause you more harm than success. Remember that the more ingredients there are, the more that product can give you harmful effects. Some irritants include ammonia, balsam, bergamot, citrus juices, and citrus oils. However, the reactions may still differ among different users with different skin types. Still, it does not hurt to watch what you put on your skin.

Skin Care Tip #66: Find Your T-Zone

Although oily skin is way better than dry skin's potential of creating irritation and wounds, it is also prone to problems such as the formation of blemishes. So if you have oily skin, try applying a toner in a T-form on your face. Try it on a horizontal line on your forehead and a vertical line down to your nose. This will reduce your chances of having acne, blackheads, and white heads.

Skin Care Tip #67: Sunscreen for Your Lips

Your lips is one of the thinly covered parts of your body. And just as much as any area of the skin, your lips deserve the care and protection that would not leave it dried, chapped, and cracked. Keep your skin from the harsh rays of the sun by investing on some sunscreen for your lips as well.

Skin Care Tip #68: Vaseline for Softer Hands

The skin on your hands may seem rough, scaly, and dry from all the working that they do. But do not fret, simply by coating your hands with Vaseline overnight while having it covered with cotton gloves, you can already wake up to softer and smoother hands.

Chapter 5 - Affordable and Easy DIY Beauty Products

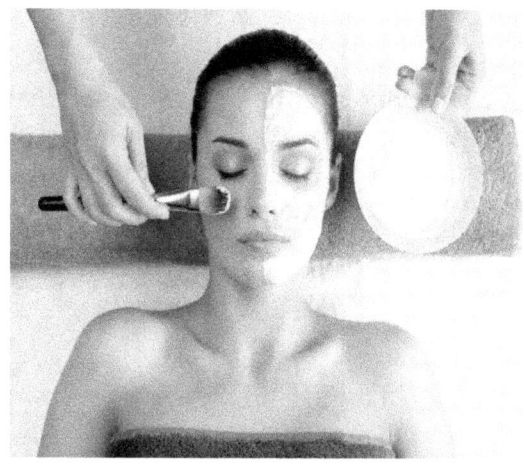

Keeping your skin healthy does not necessarily mean you have to rob off a bank or spend every single cent of your money on all those skin care products that all claim to be the number one. You can go cheap and easy on having healthier and younger-looking skin just by making your own face masks, moisturizers, and exfoliators.

You may want to go to your backyard, garden, or kitchen to discover that most of the items that you can find there could be used for keeping the health of your skin at its best state. You can use herbs, vegetables, and fruits as ingredients for natural and do-it-yourself skin care products.

So, why spend around hundreds of dollars on skin care items that you can just make at home? These are accessible and easy to do skin care products that will leave you no excuse on why you should not make them.

Skin Care Tip #69: Bask in Some Raw and Organic Honey Face Mask

Organic and raw honey is a natural skin care product that you can use for a more glowing skin. All you have to do is get a tablespoon of raw and organic honey and rub it warm on your fingertips then to your face. Spread it evenly around and then leave it for 5 to 10 minutes. Use warm water to rinse off the raw honey and pat your face dry.

Skin Care Tip #70: Try this Elbow and Knee Exfoliate and Skin Brightener

You do not have to stress your skin to exfoliate. Through natural products like an orange for example, you can exfoliate dark parts of your skin – your elbow and your knees. These thick and rough patches of skin will be softened and more moisturized by rubbing a halved orange on them and rinsing off the stickiness after. This will leave you with softer and more radiant knees and elbows with that citrus smell as well.

Skin Care Tip #71: Use a Gentle Body Scrub

For a ratio of 2:1, you may use olive oil and sea salt to make a more organic and raw body scrub with less manufactured chemicals that may only harm your skin. This cheap and easy to do body scrub will help you get rid of the dead skin cells and will help you make way for a more glowing and softer skin.

Skin Care Tip #72: Go for an All-Natural Black Head Removal

Black heads do not need heavy chemical additions just to have them removed. You can use raw and organic honey and a single lemon that is cut into wedges. Drop a few of raw honey on an open lemon wedge and rub the lemon on your face, most especially, emphasize on the areas with black heads. Then leave the mixture on your face for around 5 minutes then rinse off with cold water.

Skin Care Tip #73: Do-It-Yourself Facial Masks to the rescue

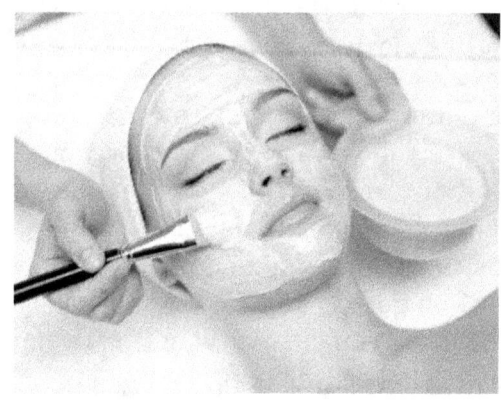

Whenever you encounter skin problems or issues, you may always resort to do-it-yourself facial masks to refresh your skin by clearing away the dead skin and getting rid of blemishes and imperfections. These facial masks need not be expensive and difficult to do. They can easily be found in your kitchen or garden. You may use fruit acids and enzymes for facial masks in order to get rid of dead skin cells and freshen up your skin.

Skin Care Tip #74: Peelings for Your Skin

You may use the inner peels of bananas and apply it on your face to serve as a natural moisturizer. Rinse it off after 15 minutes. You may also use potato peelings when your skin is puffy, avocadoes for improved complexion, and pineapple for a brighter skin. These peelings have hidden benefits to your skin that you may definitely make use of.

Skin Care Tip #75: Brown Sugar and Banana Chunk Organic Body Scrub

You can use brown or yellow banana chunks. Finely mash it up with brown sugar. You may use your fingers to have it evenly crushed and mashed. Then, shape it up with a container of your choice and have it dried.

Skin Care Tip #76: Grapefruit and Avocado in Sugar Body Scrub

This grapefruit and avocado combination is best for your skin. Grapefruits have antioxidants that protect your skin from developing skin cancer and they also contain free-radicals that can equalize your skin tone and free your skin of blemishes and wrinkles. More so, the oil contained in avocado cannot block your pores when you apply it to your skin so you are basically allowing your pores to breathe still. With the mixture of both grapefruit and avocado oil in sugar, mashed and finely stirred, you can have your own body scrub that is naturally good for your skin.

Skin Care Tip #77: Coffee and Coconut Oil in Sugar Scrub

With coffee's antioxidant powers and coconut oil's natural moisturizing prowess, this tandem could give your skin protection and better health. All you have to do is mix both ingredients smoothly and evenly and shape up to your desire until it dries.

Skin Care Tip #78: Lemon Yeast Paste

To get rid of your skin blemishes, you might want to try making this Lemon Yeast paste. You will need Brewer's yeast, 2 to 3 table spoons of lemon juice, and water. Mix all these ingredients together and apply the paste on your blemished area.

Leave it on for 10 minutes and cover it with a bandage or cloth. These ingredients can fight off the bacteria in your blemish and can cause it to be gone in just a few days.

Skin Care Tip #79: Anti-Acne Dried Basil Leaves

If you know you are actually prone to blemishes like acne, then this do-it-yourself skin care product is best for you. You will only need 2 to 3 tablespoons of dried basil herb leaves and a cup of water. Heat up your cup of water until it comes to a boil while you crush the dried basil leaves on another corner. Then pour the crushed leaves on the boiling water, turn down the fire, and allow the mixture to cool. Sift off the leaves and pour the mixture into a spray bottle. Spray the mixture on a cotton ball before you cleanse.

Skin Care Tip #80: Brandy and Peach Summer Facial Wash

In time for summer and basking under the heat of the sun, aside from some sunscreen protection, you can also use some summer facial wash for your skin. You will need a brandy and mashed peach mixed together. Apply the mixture to your face and leave it on for 20 minutes. Then rinse it off with warm water.

Skin Care Tip #81: Essential Oils for Your Feet

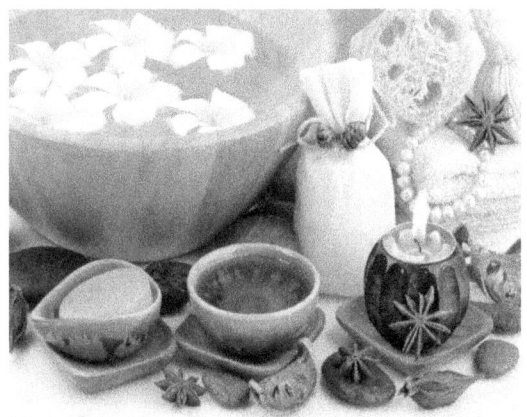

Your feet also need intensive skin care. Take good care of them by applying a few drops of essential oil on your foot bath. These oil will help smoothen and soften your feet and prevent it from cracking dry and wounding.

Skin Care Tip #82: Cocoa Butter for your Feet

The reason for smelly feet is that it is most often sweaty. To have drier feet, you may want to try this natural and easy skin care application. Smother some cocoa butter on your feet, slip into some plastic bags, and wear a pair of over-sized socks. Leave this on your feet for one night over and you will wake up with smoother, silkier, and softer skin on your feet.

Skin Care Tip #83: Oatmeal Facial Mask

Aside from having it as your day-starter meal, oatmeal also has other benefits such as its effectiveness in making the skin look younger, smoother, and more relaxed. Organic oatmeal contains less pesticide, herbicides, and GMOs so you are assured that it is less *poisonous*. More so, oatmeal is rich in amino acids that are the building blocks of protein, making your skin feel firmer and younger. All you have to do is create a pasty mixture of oatmeal and water and allow it to cool down a bit then apply it on your skin.

Skin Care Tip #84: Egg Yolk Facial Mask

Our skin's absorbent powers works well with having egg yolks as facial mask. Yolks are rich in vitamins and minerals that when you use them as facial mask and apply them to your face, your skin will absorb these nutrients directly from the fresh and natural source.

Skin Care Tip #85: Egg White Facial Mask

Eggs' dual purpose for facial masking will be of your benefit since you can also make use of the egg white as a facial mask. Compared to the egg yolk, egg whites have more protein in them which means that when you apply them to the skin, you can immediately feel it tightening. This will make your face look fresher and firmer. This natural facial mask can easily get you to let go of wrinkles and say hello to a healthier and younger-looking skin.

Skin Care Tip #86: Olive Oil Moisturizer

You may have some olive oil in your kitchen and perhaps, without your knowledge, this has benefits that can extend directly to having healthy skin. Olive oil is a good skin moisturizer since it will not clog up your pores and even allow the reduction of red spots and signs of aging on your skin with its anti-inflammatory and antioxidant properties. Simply apply olive oil on your skin and you can expect it to look and feel healthier and more vibrant.

Skin Care Tip #87: Dark Chocolate Facial Mask

Perhaps it is quite a shocking news to have dark chocolate splattered on your face to make it healthier but this facial mask works well and is even used in some ritzy spas. Dark chocolate is rich in antioxidants that can fight off the free radicals on your skin. These antioxidants can help prevent skin dehydration and drying. All you have to do is have the organic dark chocolate melted and cooled down a bit, then you may apply it on your face already.

Skin Care Tip #88: Teabags for your Eye Areas

We often neglect the areas around our eyes when we take care of our skin. But these areas are also very prone to skin problems and most especially puffing. In order to get rid of puffy areas around your eyes, you may soak two teabags in cold water and use a cotton ball or soft cloth to pat the said areas.

Skin Care Tip #89: Do not Let Stretch Marks Leave Marks Anymore

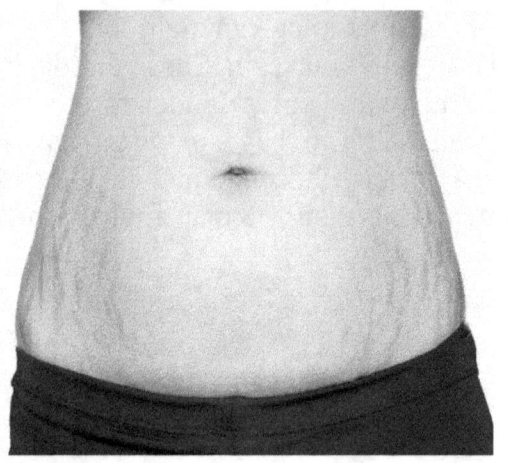

We may have stretch marks in different parts of our body — our thighs, stomachs, arms, and others, but these stretch marks do not necessarily have to leave a mark permanently because with the application of Vitamin E oil on the skin, these stretch marks could fade and you will notice it gone in a matter of weeks.

Skin Care Tip #90: Sand Body Scrub

When you are at the beach enjoying the heat of the sun, you may give yourself a body rub with the sand. This will help you exfoliate your dead skin cells. Still, do not forget to add up some sun screen.

Skin Care Tip #91: Shea Butter for Better Skin

For a smoother and youthful-looking skin, you may apply Shea Butter and rinse with warm water afterwards. This will help your skin become softer and free of blemishes.

Skin Care Tip #92: Tomato Juice Facial Mask

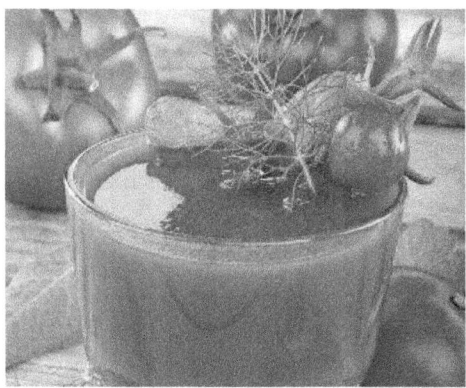

Tomatoes have high contents of acid and potassium that could naturally help you get rid of skin blemishes just by applying tomato juice on your face. Leave it on for 15 to 20 minutes then rinse with warm water afterwards.

Skin Care Tip #93: Skin Cool Down

Shrink and tighten your pores by wrapping ice or ice cubes in a soft cloth and gently pat your skin with it. For a small amount of time, this can decrease the release of sebum from your skin.

Skin Care Tip #94: Plain Yogurt Facial Mask

Yogurt can also aid you in tightening and firming your pores. Simply apply plain yogurt on your face and leave it on for around 20 minutes. Rinse your face with warm water afterwards. Do this twice every week.

Skin Care Tip #95: Papaya Paste

Papayas are usually used in making soaps that are meant to keep the skin blemish-free but even by simply applying mashed papaya on your face, it can already help you purify your skin and remove the impurities. Leave the paste on for around 20 minutes and rinse with warm water afterwards.

Skin Care Tip #96: Aloe Vera Moisturizer and Facial Mask

The juice of aloe vera can serve as a moisturizer and a facial mask. Its juice can cleanse and provide nutrients to the skin and at the same time shrink and make the pores firmer. Its moisturizing purposes also gives the skin a radiant natural glow by removing the oil and dirt from clogged pores and replacing it with a replenished look.

Skin Care Tip #97: Sweet and Salty Body Scrub

The mixture of sugar and salt are best and effective skin exfoliators. Just mix a tablespoon of brown sugar, a teaspoon of salt, and a tablespoon of honey thoroughly in a bowl. Apply this mixture on any part of your skin — whether it is you face, back, neck, or even your lips. This natural scrub is safe for your body but of course, do not forget to rinse it off with warm water afterwards.

Chapter 6- Additional Health Tips

Still, there are other factors that could affect the health of your skin – some of which involve habits that you have to engage with daily while others can be done through exercises and proper rest and stress management. And you can exercise control over these factors. Here are additional tips to keep your skin healthy.

Skin Care Tip #98: No to Excessive Sun Expose

The sun may be at its optimal strength to ruin your skin cells and increase your risk of getting skin cancer with its extreme heat in between 10 in the morning up to 2 in the afternoon. So to avoid any damage that it may cause, avoid exposing yourself directly in the sun in between these times without any protection.

Skin Care Tip #99: Dress Up for the Weather

Exposing your skin barely to the sun's harmful rays most especially during the red alert times will increase your risk of getting skin cancer and can even causing you to suffer from sunburn. So to keep this from happening, wear protective clothing that can cover your skin enough. You may also use wide-brimmed hats to keep your face from being too exposed under the sun.

Skin Care Tip #100: DO NOT Smoke

Smoking does not only affect you lungs, it also narrows down the blood vessels in the outermost layers of your skin. When these vessels are narrowed down, blood flow is decreased which means that the nutrients and oxygen could not be transmitted well to the skin. This causes the wrinkling of the skin, thus making you look way past your age.

Skin Care Tip #101: Get Enough Sleep

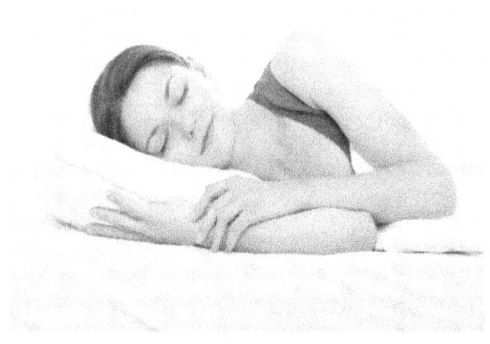

Getting a good night's rest is one of the most essential keys to a healthier looking skin. It allows the rejuvenation of cells thus making your skin look healthier and younger. A few tips to get a good quality of sleep at night is to engage in exercise or avoid heavy dinners.

Skin Care Tip #102: Own a Plant

Keeping a clean space is one of the suggested tips in having a healthier skin since it keeps off particles that may cause skin irritation. Additionally, having indoor plants in your area will refresh the air and filter it more. So you are more assured that you have a cleaner atmosphere that is almost null with toxic and irritation-causing particles.

Skin Care Tip #103: De-stress Yourself

Do not be afraid to eliminate distress from your life. Your stress inside will reflect on your skin and prevent it from living to its full blown bloom.

Skin Care Tip #104: Exercise Regularly

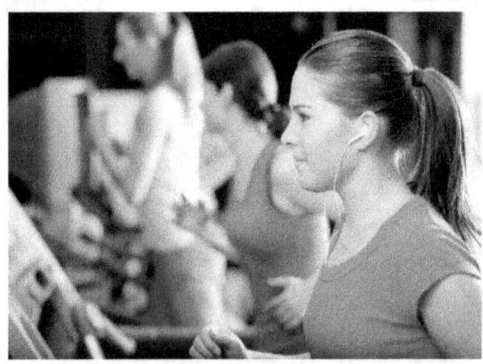

Have some time to engage in physical activities — run, job, swim, do yoga or Pilates, or just simply move around a lot. Kinetic activities will help your oxygen and nutrient circulation increase and aid in eliminating toxins from your body through sweat. In order to have a clearer and firmer skin, regular exercise is the solution.

Skin Care Tip #105: Avoid Picking your Skin

Some engage in habits or mannerisms of picking their skin when they are nervous or bored. But this act of doing so may put one into the risk of scarring and skin infection. Skin picking wounds may not always heal properly and sooner or later turn into acne.

Skin Care Tip #106: Know the Benefits of Having a Facial Massage

Facial massage may improve the circulation of blood in your epidermis. This can improve the firmness of your skin, reduce wrinkles, stress lines, as well as loosen of your facial muscles.

Skin Care Tip #107: Take Off a Steam

Steaming off can help you open up your pores to improve the circulation of blood in your epidermis and release the toxins. This is an easy skin care process that only involves a pot of water, fire, and a soft towel. Start off by boiling a pot of water.

Let the water simmer for 5 to 10 minutes under low heat then put the pot on a dry countertop or table. Place the soft towel over your head and lean your face towards the steam of the pot of water. Stay in this position for 5 minutes then rinse off with cool water afterwards.

Skin Care Tip #108: Give Your Skin Some Zen Time

Perhaps you have noticed that when you are too stressed from work, school, or even with personal problems, you start to grow pimples and acne. High levels of stress can cause your body to produce more cortisol and other hormones that could lead to breakouts of skin problems. Worse, they can also aggravate psoriasis conditions, especially if there is already an existing problem. Give yourself some time to de-stress and relax. You may take a ten-minute time out before bed for a facial mask application and allow yourself to get some rest. You need that.

Skin Care Tip #109: Lessen on Cardio

Although exercise helps in clearing the skin and making it look fresher and younger, too much time spent on cardio exercises such as running, jogging, swimming, and biking can weaken your collagens and may lead into the sagging of your skin. Limit your cardio exercises in

20 to 30 minutes instead, or do intervals instead.

Skin Care Tip #110: Avoid Tanning

With all the problems in global warming and ozone hole, you now have to think twice of basking yourself under the extreme heat of the sun. Looking tan may keep your beach vibe heaping but it also means you are closing yourself towards some harmful skin problems, most especially skin cancer. So as much as possible, avoid tanning but if you really want to, you may choose better times of the day to tan and not in between 10 in the morning to 2 in the afternoon and do not forget your sun screen.

Skin Care Tip #111: Examine your Skin

Do a monthly self-check on your skin at least once a month. Take note of the little differences or improvements. There may be some effects of the new products that you are using or new regimens that you are trying. Checking yourself every once in a while will keep you on track to achieving a healthier and more youthful-looking skin.

Skin Care Tip #112: See Your Dermatologist or Physician

Should you encounter skin problems when using certain products, do not hesitate to see a physician or dermatologist. Do not self-medicate or ignore these skin problems because in most cases, they can only get worse. Trust your physicians and dermatologists to know better and handle your problems well.

Skin Care Tip #113: It's all about the Position

If you observe your feet and ankles to be swelling, you have this red alert of knowing that you might be holding too much fluids in your system. To avoid the swelling, try other positions other than sitting. More so, reduce your sodium intake as it also adds up to the problem.

Skin Care Tip #114: Watch your Medications

If you are under medication, you might want to consider asking your doctor if the drugs you are taking could affect your skin. Some medicines like aspirin and other blood-thinners and non-condensers can have side-effects on your skin by making it bruise so easily.

There are also antibiotics and vitamins that can lead your skin to be easily burnt under the sun. Knowing the possible side effects will give you a warning on what to do. So, if you are taking these antibiotics and vitamins, you know you should take extra care of your skin especially when you know you are going to stay long under the sun.

Skin Care Tip #115: Be careful with Temporary Tattoos

As much as permanent tattoos have their risks, temporary ones share the same issues on potentially causing irritation on the skin. Henna, for example, is commonly used in making temporary tattoos but this may cause infections, inflammations, and allergic reactions. Henna is merely approved by the U.S. Food and Drug Administration as a hair dye and not as a product to be applied on the skin.

Skin Care Tip #116: Stretch Out, Bend and Break Skin Problems

Yoga is a form of mind and body exercise that will develop your full potential. It can help you with improved blood circulation, reduce inflammation, and manage the stress that has been clawing on you for days. All these benefits of yoga can give your skin a healthy and radiant glow.

Skin Care Tip #117: Keep Your Products Closer

Some may fall back and find it hard to stick to their skin care regimen. The best way is to keep these products close and visible to you so you would be reminded of your usual skin regimen. You may place your night-time products on your bedside table so before you turn off the lamp, you will get the sight of these products and then you would not have to worry about forgetting about them anymore. You may also place some of these cosmetics in your bathroom sink for easier access and more visibility or in any way that you can keep your products closer to you as a reminder.

Skin Care Tip #118: Do Not Forget to Smile

Your face is made up of muscles that create muscle memory. And one of the factors why we develop wrinkles and stress lines on our face is because of our usual expressions. These expressions leave marks on the memory of our facial muscles that when we frown most of the time, our facial skin often follows and sags as well, creating wrinkles. When we laugh and smile more often, laugh lines may be created but these lines give your face a more relaxing state.

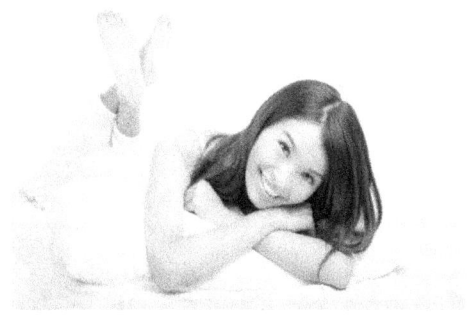

CONCLUSION

Thank you again for downloading this book!

Your skin is the biggest organ of your body that needs your huge attention and care. It serves many purposes that are necessary for our survival that if we disregard their proper care, we also disregard our survival tendencies. Putting our skin at risk also means we are putting our lives at risk since our skin does so any things for us that we should never really take for granted. They are our protective barriers, outlets for toxic wastes, body condition barometer, and comfort and pleasure source. With the given healthy skin regimens and tips, you may already start off on deciding how to approach your way of caring for your skin.

You can eat your way to a healthier skin, give it a healthy environment, use the science of cosmetics, and make your own skin care products, and relaxation and other techniques. Just make sure that you are doing all these for the sake of giving your skin the best health from inside and out.

Aside from all these tips, you will need perseverance and determination with prior safety check-ups every once in a while. Giving your skin utmost care will reflect exactly on how it will appear on the outside. But keep in mind that how you treat your skin will definitely show. Keep it healthy and it will appear to be healthy as well.

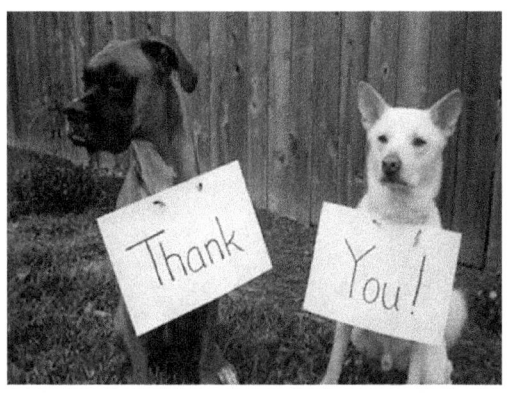

Finally, if you enjoyed this book, then I'd like to ask you for a favor, would you be kind enough to leave a review for this book on Amazon? It'd be greatly appreciated!

Click here to leave a review for this book on Amazon!

Thank you and good luck!

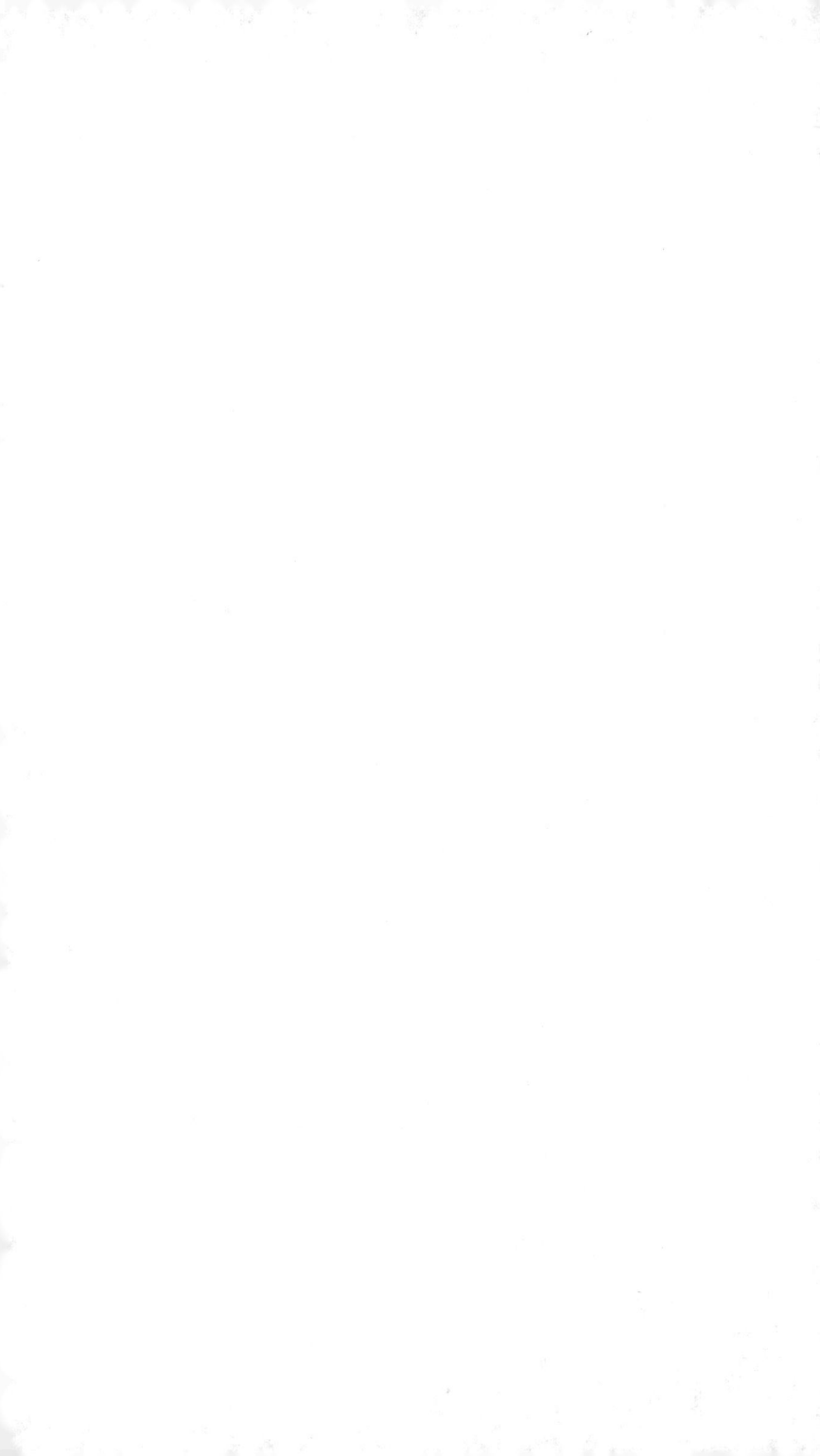

www.ingramcontent.com/pod-product-compliance
Lightning Source LLC
Chambersburg PA
CBHW071215280526
45787CB00002B/691